Not Eating!

Drop the Fork and Let the Good Times Roll

by Greg Bass

Copyright © 2016 by Greg Bass

Scripture taken from The Message. Copyright © 1993, 1994, 1995, 1996, 2000, 2001, 2002. Used by permission of NavPress Publishing Group.

THE HOLY BIBLE, NEW INTERNATIONAL VERSION®, NIV® Copyright © 1973, 1978, 1984, 2011 by Biblica, Inc.® Used by permission. All rights reserved worldwide.

DISCLAIMER: THIS BOOK DOES NOT PROVIDE MEDICAL ADVICE
The information, including but not limited to, text, graphics, images and other material contained in this book are for informational purposes only. This book is not intended to be a substitute for professional medical or mental health advice, diagnosis or treatment. Always seek the advice of your physician or other qualified health care provider with any questions you may have regarding a medical condition or treatment and before undertaking a new health care regimen, and never disregard professional medical advice or delay in seeking it because of something you have read in this book.

TABLE OF CONTENTS

FACE PLANT
HOPE!
LOOKIN GOOD?
WHERE'S WALDO?
GET UP!
GET OVER IT!
DO THIS!
NUMERO UNO
NOT THE "SECRET"
FIGHT'S NOT OVER YET
YOU GOTTA BE KIDDING ME!
HE COULD GO ALL THE WAY!
TURN OUT THE LIGHTS, THE PARTY'S OVER
LOOK OUT!
GET THAT WEAK STUFF OUTTA HERE!
ZERO TO SIXTY
ME ME ME
STEP AWAY FROM THE COOKIE!
EAT YOUR VEGETABLES!
WHAT'S YOUR PROBLEM?!
WAMMO
WAIT THERE'S MORE!
RIPPED UP LIKE A DUECE!
SMH!
KNOCK IT OFF!
WHAT THE!
GOING TO CALIFORNIA
BIG BAD WOLF
TAKE THIS JOB AND SHOVE IT!
SIRI, TAKE ME TO THE PROMISED LAND
NOTHING TO SEE HERE
THIS WILL ONLY HURT A LITTLE

FACE PLANT

It's 4am, and I'm face down in an asphalt parking lot, screaming into an oil spot. My mouth, my nose, my eyes just full-face on the ground. My arms and legs are spread out, and I'm crying out to no one in particular but hopefully to a God I'm not even sure exists.

It's pitch black in the middle of the night, and I'm spread eagled and hollering. I've ridden my bike there in the deep dark because I don't have a car anymore. I don't know what else to do or where to go so I just collapse and give up. I've sold the last of our cars, along with the trailer, and the other bikes and even the nice furniture. The savings and the 401k and the kids' college funds are long gone. And now, finally, there's nothing left to sell. I have nothing left and no money. None. I can't get a job. Shoot I can't even get a job interview. I'm about to start having to steal beer if I want to keep drowning in it. Miraculously, I'm still married but just barely. And I'm 46 years old.

It's the middle of the night, I'm double flat broke, laying face first on the cold hard ground next to a broken bicycle, and I'm screaming for God to help me.

This is the story of what happened next.

HOPE!

You should know right now that your life can finally get better. Whatever you've been struggling with, for however long, can actually get better. Almost immediately. For real.

The Bible is full of stories of people Not Eating and praying instead. Incredible miracles soon followed. My life is now full of those stories too.

I call it Not Eating, rather than calling it fasting, because I don't want anyone to get the wrong impression. If you've heard about fasting from people rather than from the stories in the Bible, you might think you can fast from chocolate or naps or Facebook or trashy TV shows. But fasting in the Bible, in other words the kind of fasting that can change your life, is Not Eating and then praying instead. So I call it Not Eating instead of calling it fasting.

I didn't know anything about Not Eating a few years ago but I was a dang expert in intransigent problems. I knew all about soul killing, life sucking problems that just wouldn't get better, but could always get worse. You may have run into some of these problems yourself, who knows. Marriage problems, money problems, friend problems, kid problems, food problems, health problems, drinking problems.

I had them all doubled over, shaken up, and coughed out. You don't end up chewing asphalt in the dark because it's all good.

Then through a series of events that I'll elaborate on a little later, I will just say God made it pretty dang clear to me that I was supposed to Not Eat and I was supposed to ask my wife Susan to Not Eat with me. So I did that. And she said yes.

Let me tell you that what I'm about to tell you is just about us. You may only have to do it for one day. Probably.

We were going to Not Eat for three days and then I would ask God to save us. Something happened during those three days and we realized we weren't ready to stop. So we kept Not Eating for 21 days. No food. No juice. No supplements. Just prayer. And water. That right then was the beginning of the second half, the better half, of my life here on earth.

Over the next year, Susan and I went on two more 21 day Not Eats, three 7 day Not Eats, and a few other shorter Not Eats. Over a 13 month period, we didn't eat for a total of about 100 days. And God saved us and totally transformed our family.

I realize from telling the story enough now, that if you don't know me or even if you do, you might think I am making this up. For the record, I am not making this up. It is true. But please please please do yourself a favor, and don't miss out on how your life can be transformed for the better based on whether you believe me or not.

I'm not asking you to believe me, because it's true no matter what. My job is not to convince you of what God did in my life but, instead, to tell you how to Not Eat, let you know what to expect, and then pray that you try it for yourself. Don't have faith in me and my story. Try having enough faith in the Lord to Not Eat for a while and see what happens. Even if you don't have enough faith, try it anyway. I was NOT all faithful in the beginning, but I was desperate.

Turns out, desperate was enough.

You definitely, Most definitely, don't have to do what we did. You don't have to quit eating for weeks on end. But if you're desperate enough in your life to try Not Eating, even for one day, in hopes that there may be some help ready to come to you, please keep reading. That one day may be the first day of the rest of your life, transformed.

LOOKIN GOOD?

I want you to know that I work out all the time and I always have. I also eat healthy foods and have tried so, so many different diets.

This book is not about that. All the exercise in the world and all the healthy eating never changed my life from the inside out.

Once I found out about Not Eating, taking my mind off food completely and putting it on God instead, my life started a radical transformation.

That's what this book is about.

I still work out and eat healthy because it makes me feel good and look okay for an old dude. But that is not what this book is about.

My wife, Susan Bass, went through all of this with me, side by side. The stories and ideas here come from our shared life. But the words in this book all come from me. You can't blame her for what follows. So back off bub.

WHERE'S WALDO?

About this whole Not Eating thing, I know what you're thinking right off the bat because I think it too every time I think about what you're thinking about. Here it is:

Not Eating? Not going to do it. No food? No way. I can't do it. It's going to suck. What about lunch? What about dinner? What about breakfast? And shoot, I'm kind of hungry right now. And then you go eat.

Every person who ever Not Ate thought the same thing before they did it too. Here's some people who did Not Eat even though they wanted to eat: Moses, Jesus Christ, King David, Elijah, St. Paul, Gandhi, Cesar Chavez. And me, Greg Bass.

One of these things is not like the other. So funny. But seriously, my name is in there too, even though I am ridiculous. If you knew me, you'd know it's not because I'm in the same high moral league as great people from history. My name is in there because Anybody can Not Eat and get a miracle, even if that person is a big screwup. Like me. Or, perhaps, like you.

Listen up: do you know what it's like to be wracked with guilt? Or immobilized by sadness? Or seething with anger? Or addicted to something stupid?

Now can you remember what it's like to be a little hungry? I can. Given the choice between short-term hunger and lifelong regret, I choose the hunger. Because it's only physical and doesn't last. Shame can drown your soul until you are dead. Arguments - oh my Lord arguments! - can wreck your life until you have no life left. But skipping a few meals will fly by. And if you do it right, you just might find some real freedom. Interested?

If you start studying fasts in the Bible, or just finish reading this little book, you will see that the people who've Not Eaten are like a Who's Who of the Bible. There are so many stories of Not Eating told over centuries in there, that you may be surprised to find out Every story has this one thing in common:

Virtually every story that begins with Not Eating ends with an amazing victory. The chains get broken. Lives are spared. Cities are saved. An entire race of people gets the victory. Enemies are defeated. Families are restored. Sicknesses healed. All because they Stopped Eating and started praying.

The captive in your life can be released, even if the captive is you, and you think you already got life without parole.

I can attest to it in my life. And I'm not holy holy, I'm not goody two shoes, I'm not apple pie and butterflies. But I tried this Not Eating thing, over and over, even though truthfully I had my doubts, and wow did things get better.

So whether you put your trust in the Bible, or you seek empirical proof of success, these methods are for you.

GET UP!

What you are reading is a kind of kick-starter: a how-to manual. This is such a short book, it's not even a book. Maybe a booklet. There's a reason, and it's not because I'm lazy.

You are supposed to get going. Just read it and do it. Rather than read some, and read some more, and discuss it in a small group, and then watch the DVD.

Of the writing of books, there is no end. Too much reflection and study makes you weary. That is in the book of Ecclesiastes. Solomon predates Nike.

This is not a book of theology. Everything I learned about fasting I learned from reading the Bible and then just doing what the people in it did.

If you want to read more about Not Eating later, here's a few places where you can find stories in the Bible. Don't go there now. Esther, Matthew, Acts, Exodus, Jonah, Nehemiah, Kings, Ezra, Mark, Daniel, Isaiah. Most of the heavy hitters in the Bible did it. You know, like Jesus, Moses,

Paul. The list goes on. But this book is not some exhausting and exhaustive list of fasts. Just turn the page and get on with it.

GET OVER IT!

Not Eating is not going to kill you. It may just save your life. It saved mine. Actually God saved my life. Not Eating was just the way it happened.

Don't freak out about Not Eating for 100 days in one year. All you have to do is Not Eat on One day and seek the Lord instead and see what happens.

You've probably eaten every day of your life, and it hasn't saved you so far. So just try Not Eating for a day.

If it goes for a second day or third day or even longer, you deal with those days when they get there. Today's challenges are enough for today. No use worrying about tomorrow because that doesn't fix anything.

Here are some possible titles for this book:

Save your marriage, by Not Eating.

Quit drinking as a crutch, by Not Eating.

Get a good job, by Not Eating .

Look younger, feel happy, lose weight, by Not Eating.

Find your soulmate, by Not Eating.

Discover true friendship, by Not Eating, .

Find God's plan for your life, by Not Eating.

Heal disease, by Not Eating.

Save your people from destruction, by Not Eating.

All these things have happened in my family by Not Eating and truly seeking God in those times instead. Problems that were just never going to go away are gone now. GONE. Where there was no hope there have been complete breakthroughs.

Do you want that in your life? Then follow this book, which is just a condensed version of the Not Eating stories of the Bible, with some helpful hints thrown in. I say again: Do you want breakthrough?

Some people would rather die than try Not Eating. The only difference between them and me is that I finally got so desperate that I would rather die than keep living a life with no hope. I thank God that he grabbed me and told me to try Not Eating. So I did. And my wife did with me.

And God saved our marriage. And God saved our family. And God gave us awesome work for our hands. And God healed our bodies. And God healed our troubled souls. And God gave us true friendships. God saved us from certain destruction.

And now it's your turn.

You probably never talk about Not Eating, even if you go to church every week, plus a Bible study, and a small group, plus watch two preachers on TV. You probably have no idea just how prominent Not Eating is in the Bible. How would you? Nothing empties the pews or drops the ratings faster than telling people to give up eating.

If a new Not Eating movement started, a Not Eating Sucks countermovement would grow faster, with bumper stickers, and billboards, and callers to talk shows. It's like the most frightening thing you can suggest to many people.

But Not Eating is a pretty big deal in the Bible, and it pretty much always ends in incredible miracles in the favor of those who did the Not Eating.

So if you're looking for a miracle, maybe you should listen up.

I could start telling you about all the amazing things that can happen in your life if you were to just Not Eat.

But no matter how many miracles I relate, from ancient manuscripts or from the life of Greg, I'm concerned you won't even be paying attention because all you're hear in the back of your mind the whole time is this little running dialogue:

I can't Not Eat. It sounds great, but I'll never be able to do it. I like food too much. Blah blah, blah. Blah blah blah.

Well let me say this to the back of your mind for just a second, respectfully:

Bull crud.

I like food as much as you do, probably more. I get hungry as much as you do, probably more. I've been a world class eating machine. And I didn't think I could do it, but I did. And here's how.

It gets easier over time. I have to tell you how the story ends, sorry. The more you Not Eat and the longer you Not Eat, the less hungry you are (at least for the first 3 weeks - I know that sounds ridiculous, but we're just talking about 1 day for you, okay? Don't get your shorts bunched up). After a while, it's no biggie. It's like anything else you quit doing, except easier because you know you'll start up again soon enough. So if you've ever quit smoking or drinking or smoking crack, this is way easier because it's only temporary.

If you are following along at home, you might want to know just exactly what you're supposed to do. Read on son.

DO THIS!

So here's what'll happen when you're Not Eating: as soon you begin Not Eating, on that first morning, even before you would normally feel hunger, you will start thinking about food. Thoughts of eating may shoot at your brain like little laser beams, pew pew pew. It's time to eat, pew pew pew. You must be hungry, pew pew pew. Whenever you think of food, stop right then and pray. Every time you think of eating, ask God not only take away your hunger but to fix whatever you're Not Eating for in the first place.

Super Duper disclaimer: I am not trying to save your soul. I am trying to teach you how to get the change you've been dying to get. Keep that in mind during this paragraph. Here's another thing you should start doing on day one: When you are Not Eating food, eat the word of God instead (I understand that for some people that sounds just ridiculous - I don't really give a hoot, comprende?) Read the Bible. Dive into it with that hunger you would have turned toward food on a normal day. Jesus is right in there, and he is the bread that will satisfy and heal you, whether you buy into it right now or not.

Again, I'm not trying to save your soul. I'm trying to help you be free of whatever ails you. So pray – that's you talking to God. And read the word – that's God talking to you. Don't worry about if you are doing it right. Just read it. I believe God wants to talk to you, and he doesn't usually use bumper stickers. And even if you don't know if you believe in the whole Jesus and God thing, read the Bible during you're Not Eating time anyway.

Just try it. I didn't believe any of it for a long time myself. In fact I was one of the most skeptical people on earth, only out skepticized by my wife. And I'm the one now telling you all this. And all because I was desperate enough to try anything because my life was such a pile.

I was not all in on faith. I would have never made it that way. It's only because of what God started doing in my life. Miracles started showing up in my life in ways I could not explain or deny, over and over and over. Until finally I had no choice but to believe. So whether you believe or not, just try this Not Eating thing.

NUMERO UNO

So you know what happens first you wake up knowing you're not going to eat: all you think about is food. This too shall pass. When you think of eating, just don't eat. In fact, when you think about food on that day, don't eat but pray instead. This book is about Not Eating and praying instead. So on that day you will be praying all day. It's good for you.

Don't get ahead of yourself. Don't think about how you're Not going to eat for the whole day. Don't unnecessarily freak yourself out. You don't have to Not Eat for a whole day all at once, just one Not bite at a time.

Here's what else to expect: you are going to have so much extra time on your hands. Taking your mind off of your own eating and putting it in the kingdom of heaven somehow has a multiplying effect on the hours in your day. You can take a walk and read the Bible and do some gardening and play some cards and still have time leftover. We even started watching the food channel on TV at night as some sort of sick joke on ourselves. Really. No kidding. Even if you still make food for other people, you will still have way more free time. Don't ask me how. It's some sort of negative reverse synergism.

So you're going to get through short periods of wanting food by praying. You're going to read the Bible. You're going to stay busy. And you're just Not going to eat. It's only one day. You won't die. You're going to be hungry but you'll go to sleep and wake up the next day and you will have done it.

NOT "THE SECRET"

Here's the one piece of information in this book about Not Eating that I did not learn from the Bible, but instead from hands-on experience.

A secret, if you will. If you want to make your time of Not Eating a happy time, or at least a little less sad time, go buy these three things before it starts. Sugar free gum, a jar of pickles, and diet Dr Pepper.

When you are Not Eating, especially for extended periods, you will quickly miss the act of chewing. Seriously. Pop in some sugar free gum and your chewing fix is fixed. And when you start to feel a little hungry or grumpy, swig some pickle juice. You may call BS right now, but just you wait. Get you some salty garlicky vinegar, and you'll be good to go. Your brain may just keep working a little. And diet Dr. Pepper? It's just delicious. All three of these things have one thing in common, though, and that is they all have zero calories.

And please drink water. I know there's a few examples of people giving up both food And water. But we did not quit drinking water. Not Eating was what I was called to. Not drinking water would be above my pay grade. I am not recommending it. Try Not Eating food - that should be enough fun in itself.

So you are drinking water, but you are Not Eating. So you can't be drinking calories. This ain't no juice fast, just a fast. No smoothies either, you tricky little people. No calories, ok? Just Not Eating and praying instead. It won't kill you, but it might just save you instead.

Here's another little secret. The first day is the hardest. Wait wait wait, I can hear you say I'm not sure I can get through that one day, much less more than one day. I get it. I do. You may recall that my wife and I did our first Not Eat and that ended up lasting 21 days. I would never have started it at all had I known it would go for that long.

But as it happened, God started doing miracles in my family and we just wanted to keep going. We ended up Not Eating for a total of 100 days over the next year. Not because we didn't like food, but because we loved what started happening in our lives. More on that a little later.

We actually used to look forward to our next Not Eat. That's a true statement, even though here's a few of my favorite things: Boston cream pie, brisket, tri-tip, garlic bread, extreme Moose tracks ice cream. I love food. And yet I couldn't wait to Not Eat it.

Why? Because somehow by putting all my focus on the God of Angel armies, He started fixing me. Freeing me. Blessing me in ways I couldn't even imagine. He saved me. He saved my family. And He will do the same for you if you seek Him out with all you've got.

FIGHT'S NOT OVER YET

So on the second day, you might just wake up and say: I'm going to stick with this Not Eating a little while longer.

Day 2 will be a little easier. You're not going to be quite as hungry. You're not going to think about food quite as much. But you should keep praying like nobody's business. You should read even more of the Bible.

Or do some gardening and mindfully meditate if you want. There's basically two kinds of people who might be reading this. One, you're the kind of person who looks to the Bible for direction and help. Two, you're the kind of person who doesn't go looking in the Bible for answers, but you need help with something big in your life. I was more like that when I started. I needed so much help. My faith in the Bible only grew after the miracles in my life started piling up.

So just try it, whoever you are and wherever you're coming from. It works. I promise. That's all you need to know. I can't explain it, even though I would like to. And once again it doesn't matter to me one bit if you believe my story, our story, about fasting with no food and no calories and no juice - no nothing like that - for 100 days in one year. But

I will tell the story because some of you are going to try it, and some of you are going to be saved, and I don't even know you. And to tell you the truth, to tell you the hard truth, I don't really care. But I feel compelled to do this, compelled like I have no other choice but to do it, so I'm doing it. I don't really want to put myself out there as some person who says Do this or Do that because the Bible says it. I've seen people say those kinds of things for mean-spirited or dumb or selfish or any number of weird reasons that turned me off and yet, now I'm doing it. So the jokes on me. Ha ha.

Here's another thing. Don't tell people that you're Not Eating. Did you hear that? Don't tell people that you're Not Eating. Why? Well, Jesus said not to, if that matters to you. Or if you just care about what works: once people know you're Not Eating, they are going to rapid fire spit out a rat a tat a tat line of discouraging words, all from a place where they Don't know anything but they Think they know everything.

People are going to talk you out of it. They're going to say bunch of scary stuff. I promise you this, right upfront, they don't know diddly squat.

They'll tell you that your body will pass out, your brain will shut down, and snakes might just fall from the sky, all if you Don't Eat. Everyone will tell you that. And 100% of them have never done it.

Let me tell you something: I freaking did it. My wife did it. And if I could give you a glimpse of my life before and after, you would freaking do it too. You don't need your trainer, your mom, your friend, or anybody else talking you out of it. Good lord you've probably already tried that stuff that they said would work and it's probably not working and that's why you're here (legal disclaimer: tell your doctor and get her or his approval first, ok?).

You are not Burning the flag, okay? You're just Not Eating. I'm going to tell you what I read in the Bible and then tried myself. Not Eating won't kill you. It just may save you.

So just don't tell anybody, okay? Unless of course they're going to fast with you. Oops, I mean Not Eat and pray instead with you.

Some of the Not Eats in the Bible were by one person alone, but, as we will see, some were by large groups. At least one was by a whole city. So feel free to enlist your people to Not Eat with you. Ramp up your sales skills. If you're having marriage problems, for instance, Not Eat with your spouse.

One more thing: I have to tell you that it says in the Bible (actually Jesus said it, so it's a pretty big deal if you're into that kind of thing) that if you fast in secret, God will reward you openly. And a reward from the Lord is pretty awesome. I've seen it firsthand. Trust me, you want some of that.

Great news from day 2; you won't be as hungry as Day 1. So you might just decide to keep going, who knows?

Again with the secrets. I mentioned this earlier in a spill the beans so you wouldn't get discouraged and quit too early moment: It gets easier as you go along. Instead of getting harder because it's longer since you've eaten, it gets a little easier as you adjust. Now you may still miss chewing just as much, so feel free to chomp on that sugar free gum. Did you hear what I said? It gets a little easier every day.

YOU GOTTA BE KIDDING ME

So let's just say you make it to Day 3. Prepare yourself, you might get a little grumpy on day three. You might get a little stupid. On our first Day 3, my wife and I Neanderthal-argued in grunts about who knows what. Clear thinking and a calm disposition were nowhere to be found. They were replaced with a shivering cold. On Day 3, you are going to need a sweater. Take hot showers and stay out of each other's way.

Because most likely, at this point if you're still Not Eating it's because you decided to Not Eat for three days. It is a common number for Not Eating in the Bible. So all you have to do is Not Eat until bedtime, and then wake up and it's Day 4. Get ready for the big day.

HE COULD GO ALL THE WAY!

Are you ready for this? Here's what happens on Day 4.

Surprise! Your hunger is gone. I mean you are not hungry anymore. And you feel pretty normal. The grumpies are gone. The stupids are gone. And the hunger is just gone. It happened to both of us multiple times. So on Day 4, rather than eating, we decided to just keep going. It's true that we were desperate. But it's also true that it got a little easier. Our lives - get this - had not – I said not - been miraculously transformed. Yet. So we kept Not Eating. For 21 days. I can tell you from first hand experience that neither one of us was hungry after that throughout the remaining 21 days.

The Big Reveal:

What I'm telling you dear brothers and sisters is you can Not Eat and pray for 21 days and you will not be hungry most of that time. If you are putting your mind and your spirit in good places along the way. Now, if you just don't eat to lose weight I cannot tell you what will happen. But it sounds like a diet and diets fail. Not Eating wins. People who don't eat and pray instead win and the last time I looked this still 'Merica - where I live at least - and in 'Merica we love winning, ha ha. Fist bump. Boom.

So something else happened on the fourth day, at least the first time that we did this. I woke up on Day 4 with a black eye. Nothing had happened to my eye the night before. Now mind you, I had woken up many times in my life with black eyes. I grew up in the 70s and 80s in Waco, Texas as an angry little guy with a chip on my shoulder, and hence forth the list of people who have given me a black guy reads like the guest list to my high school reunion. But, dear reader, I had not been in a fight on night three. I looked into it using my trusty googler and it turns out my liver was detoxing. I'd been drinking a little beer every day for two decades and then, after everything really fell apart - for a couple of years - I'd been drinking a lot of beer. Mucho cerveza, por favor. I wanted to stop, but I couldn't. It made everything worse, but I couldn't shake it. Shoot I had been binge drinking since before I had a driver's license, and I had gotten into so much trouble that I will not embarrass my people even now by giving you all the details. Let's just say I had been interested in deep trouble many times in my younger life, and most of it was because I had been liquored up.

That's what I call a persistent plague. They don't call them spirits for nothing. It's not going to be some little guy in a red suit and a tiny pitchfork standing on the wrong shoulder telling you to kick kittens. Whatever plagues you will come in disguise. Mine came as a party. Then as relaxation and stress relief. Then as escape. I prayed and prayed for deliverance but never got it.

Just like when Jesus' disciples prayed for the boy with seizures but nothing happened. And then Jesus prayed, and the boy was healed. Jesus told his people: This type can only be healed by prayer and fasting.

Long story short, my body detoxed during that first Long Not Eating. And my cravings for beer, my desire to use it in unhealthy ways, disappeared forever and never came back. It has been five years now. I tell you about it now because it's an easy thing to point out and say look at this: Not Eating and praying instead healed me of something that I could never be healed of no matter how many programs or meetings I went to, or books I read, or even prayers I tried.

Some things can only be healed by prayer and Not Eating. It's true.

And that's how we did Not Eat for 21 days the very first time we tried it.

TURN OUT THE LIGHTS, THE PARTY'S OVER

One of the main things that happens when you Stop Eating to put new focus on God by reading the word and praying instead is this: you start to become acutely aware of the thoughts running in the background of your brain.

Look out.

Something about the process doesn't actually clear your mind but it does slow it down and bringing out in the open for you to check out. Let me tell you that those thoughts, once you realize how prevalent they are in your head without you even having known that they were there before, may scare the bejeezus out of you.

After you haven't eaten in a while, on purpose, you probably will start to catch some thoughts running around the back of your skull. Thoughts that may kind of suck. Like: I'm a loser. My wife's going to leave me. I've got no real friends because I'm a big jerk. You know, screw that flippin dude; I hate him. I'm never going to be successful because I'm such an f-up. What a fat ugly piece of crap I am. No wonder I got abandoned. I should just die. Everybody'd be better off if I was dead and not screwing up their lives. Just die already. You angry scared little chicken.

Maybe you start noticing something like that, maybe not so harsh, or maybe harsher, running on an endless loop in the back your brain.

It happened to me. It wasn't pleasant at first, but you have to be aware of it so you can truly know what you are up against. Then you can ask God to start healing you from it.

And there might be some problems, angry outbursts for instance, that you could go to counseling and read books and pray about all you wanted and still get no real relief. But you could Not Eat and then slowly start to see what was running through your head to cause them. And then pray and be healed. It happened to me. Finally the relief I'd prayed and worked for with no luck. And it could suddenly be mine just by skipping a few meals? It really, actually worked.

Really, with all this Not Eating stuff, what the heck is going on? I don't know. Truly don't. But I do know it's real. It works. I certainly wouldn't be exposing myself to look like a kook once again if the stuff didn't work. Don't leave me hanging out here. Try it yourself so you can get some relief. This is going to be YOUR story.

LOOK OUT!

This is kind of the good news, bad news section: I've seen people fast for one day and be totally healed. They are just walking through their life, constantly plagued by a grown child who has gone to the dark side, or failed relationships because they can't control their anger, or one of a million other ailments, and they just can't ever seem to get better. And then they Not Eat for one day, and, boom, the chains fall off. And they're totally healed.

I can't stand those people.

But I've also seen it take longer. Sometimes way longer. Susan and I got to the end of our three day fast and we were more peeled than healed, our family was not saved, and the little devil on my shoulder was just laughing at me and poking me in the neck with his pitchfork. Like a boss. Like my boss. And so we just kept Not Eating. And that is how we ended up Not Eating for 21 days the first time. No food. No calories for three weeks. Because our desperation had not subsided.

And then we had to keep repeating it, on and off, for a year. My river of trouble was both wide and deep, friends.

To this day we still Not Eat and pray instead sometimes. But it's usually for just a day now. Before the wheels fall off, not after.

You may be a one-timer, a ten-timer, or a life-timer. I don't know. You may have to go through this Not eating and praying thing more than once to get your relief. Maybe it happens immediately for you, maybe not. I do know it can help you get rid of things that no amount of prayer on its own can get rid of. See, problems can be way trickier than just beer. Maybe you're plagued by feelings of rejection. Maybe you get angry all the time. Maybe you are filled with regret. Maybe you fight with your spouse all the time. Or maybe you're overwhelmed by anxiety and, no matter how much you pray, it won't get better. Maybe you need to Stop Eating and Start praying and Watch God work.

GET THAT WEAK SAUCE OUTTA HERE!

This is a good place to do a fake excuses breakout session. Here's some fake excuses you might hear from someone or tell yourself:

I can't fast because I've got to make food for my kids. Well, we fasted while our sons were both on the water polo and swim teams and each eating almost 10,000 calories per day. No joke. We just kept going to Costco and cooking in bulk. And I kept grilling, literally, 30 to 35 pounds of meat per week.

Another fake excuse: I have to move around too much. I can't Not Eat because I will pass out or get lightheaded or I just need calories to live. Again, I say bull crud. We actually continued to work out during our fasts. I'm not saying I did double crossfit sessions each day. But I did do some running and weight lifting almost every day while we were Not Eating. And Susan did the same.

Here's another fake excuse: I have to think too much, or I have to much to do. You will be okay. You really will. It is not the end of the world.

And one more for fun: I can't Not Eat because I have to go to business lunches. Here's a little secret. Once people's food comes to the table, they lose all interest in what you do with your food. So order some loose food that you can move around on the plate. And then stick it in a to-go box with a made up excuse of your choosing. Drink mucho diet Dr. Pepper and get refills. Activity is all you really need.

And here's something very important, mentioned in passing earlier. You cannot fast from TV. You can't fast from chocolates. You can't fast from afternoon naps. You can't fast from speeding through school zones, leaving the light on, or what ever else turns you on. Don't believe that nonsense. Let me tell you that is not fasting. Fasting is Not Eating. Not Eating. It is Not Eating. That is what it says in the Bible. That's what's going to get you your results. Don't bother fasting from anything else because it is a big waste of time and you'll make us look bad with your silliness.

ZERO TO SIXTY

One more thing, hold on, remember how I've told you before don't tell anybody that you're fasting? Well, if you go on a really long fast, I'm assuming that you broke that rule. Maybe you told somebody from your church who seemed like they might know something that could help you. Remember, they probably don't. I heard more nonsense about fasting from other Christians than from anybody else, even though the stories are all their (my) book.

They might tell you how careful you have to be about what you eat when you finally break your fast. It doesn't matter that they never did it themselves. They heard somebody sometime say something scary about fasting, and now they want to scare you too, for your own good, don't you know.

Dropping bombs like church moms. Like you have to eat soft food or yogurt or pre-chewed cud or some other ridiculousness. Let me tell you that's not anywhere in the Bible. But here's what is: fasts in the Bible are often broken by celebration feasts. I broke my first fast after 21 days with a double cheeseburger hot off the grill at a graduation party. It was

So amazingly delicious that I might just drop the mic and drive to In-N-Out right now.

ME ME ME

I mentioned that after 21 days of Not Eating we realized all was not better. Bummer. In fact, it may have looked worse because I had started to see just how messed up everything was. So I had Not Eaten for three weeks. And I felt worse. Not much of a sales pitch, I understand. Let me give you a glimpse of what happened later. We got just enough of a release during that first time to want to do it again.

And by the way, and I hate to even mention this because it's a secondary benefit for sure, but I lost weight. A bunch of weight. Weight I never regained. All that beer drinking, fast food scarfing down, sitting around waiting to croak weight just disappeared and never came back. Thirty pounds of it. And I have never gained that back. And years have gone by. I know losing weight and keeping it off is like the American dream, but I am telling you about something way greater than a diet.

I needed a lot of deliverance still, so along with my wife, I Not Ate again and then again. We never started by thinking we were going to Not Eat for longer than three days. We'd start a Not Eat and wait until it was time to stop.

And somehow the good Lord kept telling us to keep going so we just kept going. We did two more 21 day Not Eats. We did three 7 day Not Eats. We did multiple 3-day Not Eats. All in all that was 100 days with no food over the next 13 months. That's not counting the 21 day all vegetable diet we squeezed in the middle of all that. Now Jesus was before my time so I couldn't see him do it, only read about it. But, if eye witness testimony is important to you, I personally witnessed my wife go 40 days in a row without a drop of food or calories of any kind, liquid or otherwise. Call me to the stand and I will testify.

That was more extreme than you need, most of you. Right now let me just say I was totally desperate during those times. Maybe, most likely, you're not as messed up as I was. So you may not have to do what I did. That's between you and your Lord. I'm not sure anyone has ever stopped eating for 100 days in one year, at least not when there was plenty of good food around. And on purpose. But we did. Again I don't care if you don't believe me.

The only thing I brag about is that now after this journey I have a little understanding and knowledge of the Lord, at least in this area. This book is meant to take all the stories of Not Eating and put them in one, easy to read, place. I'm not adding anything to the Book; I'm just compiling it so you can check it out easily.

One big problem I have with myself is: Jesus says do this all in secret and yet here I am writing a book about it. How ridiculous is that? But like Jake and Elwood Blues, I'm on a mission from God. The same Lord that saved me will now not let me be until I finish this book. It might only be to save one person, who knows. I really, really don't like books about the Bible, when you could just be reading the actual Bible instead. Now I'm writing just such a book. Ha ha. Another joke on me.

This story is true. And, get this, we got totally transformed. If total transformation sounds good to you, Stop eating and start praying. And we are kind of the reigning world champions of Not Eating and praying, but not by our own doing that's for sure. But we did learn a little about it, so I'm going to tell you a little bit, just a little bit, of what happened to us after all that Not Eating and praying instead.

The market crashed. My company shut down. My industry disappeared. And we were stuck in a little town surrounded by open land and open sea. We eventually lost everything. All our money and assets. Everything was dying around us. Even the yard and the grass was nothing but a sandy gopher pile of stinging nettles and not much else. I couldn't get a job. I was lying and hiding about the money and then drinking in shame.

But during this time my wife started reading and reading and reading the Bible, hour upon hour, day upon day, month upon month. She had a crazy idea that she would read it for herself, instead of see what they said in Bible study or in a sermon or on the radio and, although this is not her story, I will at least say she began to be transformed. So much so that I wanted in on it. So I began trying to follow in those steps. But it didn't really work. For me, it wasn't taking. During this time, it might shock you, but it shouldn't, we were actively going to church. I was in a men's group early one morning and the janitor met me in the hallway and told me that he and his wife watched a movie about Esther from the Bible. In it, Esther fasted to get the king to save her people. And so he and his wife fasted, and it saved their marriage, and she was like a different person after that. They had been on rocky ground before and now, years later, they were good and had remained good no matter what troubles they faced along the way.

In the next week another guy told me about how his uncle had a deadly form of cancer and joined a study with 1500 other people that had it. His uncle had fasted and prayed only for other people. He was the only one in the study who survived.

And then I kept getting this word in the Bible about fasting to undo heavy burdens, break every chain, let the prisoners go, feed the hungry. In fact, it came up so many times I started just referring to it as: free the captives.

I started wondering if God was telling me to fast in some God way that I had not really experienced before, so I went to church library to look for books about fasting. I did not know it yet but would soon find out that the Bible is full of stories of fasting. I found one old book on fasting and opened it up. There was a chapter titled Free the Captives. Just to be sure I looked up in my Bible. And the passage I had been turning to never specifically says free the captives. Those were just my words that I had used to summarize the passage that I'd seen over and over again. And now those words, free the captives, were staring back at me from a musty old book with a library card showing it hadn't been checked out since the 50s. For real though.

So I decided to fast. It was less of a decision and more of me just saying, enough already God, I'll do it. I'll fast to free the captives. I can tell you with the utmost certainty that I did not yet know that the captives were us. I was prisoner number one. And I didn't even know I was wearing stripes.

I only knew one story on fasting and that was Esther, so I looked it up in the Bible. I can tell you that even though I had gone to church for years off and on, I was surprised to find that there was a book of Esther in the Bible. Who knew?

Esther was secretly an orphan would become queen. Her husband the king had an evil assistant Haman who sent out an order that all Jews must be exterminated. So Esther went to her uncle Mordecai and said she and her people would fast and asked Mordecai if he and his people would fast with her. And after three days she would go to the King and ask him to save the Jews.

It worked. Not only did the king save the Jews and kill the evil Haman, but he also gave awesome blessings to Mordecai and Esther. It's a short book. You should read it. So I went to Susan, got down on my knees and said: I'm going to fast. If you will fast with me, I will go to the Lord after three days and ask him to save our family. Because I didn't know much, but I knew my people were in grave danger. Susan said yes, she would fast with me. And so that's how it all started. Now to the good part.

It's not the end of the world. You are not going to die. You're just going to Not Eat and pray instead. You're going to eat the word instead of eat the food. It's not horrible like you think.

As I write this today, a few years later, I'm sitting at the kitchen table in our new home, looking at a panoramic view of the Pacific ocean six blocks away.

Susan has become an amazing artist working on her MFA, even though four years ago, she wasn't an artist at all. I have a thriving Medicare insurance business. Our yard is blooming with Birds of Paradise and Bougainvillea and palm trees and roses and banana plants and flowers and green grass everywhere. Our sons are both about to graduate from Cal Poly San Luis Obispo with engineering and statistics degrees, and have great jobs already lined up when they graduate. And our beautiful daughter is on the high school water polo team which just won the C.I.F. Championship in California.

But, more importantly, we have a little knowledge and understanding of God. That's not some fuzzy concept. It is everything. All other good things in our life start at that fountain.

All three of our growing children have witnessed firsthand the amazing transformation of our family. They have seen us Not Eat, and they have seen God work miracles, and they know that the Lord is real.

And I have seen each one of them Not Eat and pray instead to get help in an area that was more than they could handle.

Our marriage is the best it's ever been. My wife and I have a relationship that is so much better than it's ever been before. I'm not perfect yet, but she's working on it. Ha ha, just checking to see if she reads this far.

I have been released from raging anger, crippling hopelessness, smoking, depression, feelings of abandonment, worthlessness, nagging unbelief, and critical skepticism. And I have seen others close to me get the same new freedoms.

We Stopped Eating, prayed instead, and the Lord freed us from our captivity. Now that's what I'm talking about.

STEP AWAY FROM THE COOKIE!

If you want to Not Eat so you can lose weight, forget about it. For real. Even if you say you're Not Eating for some other reason, but you're secretly, in your heart where it matters, doing it to get skinny, just don't bother. It won't work. Or it won't last. And you'll still have your real problems. And you'll make it look bad to someone else who might be thinking about doing it. And so they will just stay in their hole and perish. And then you'll go to the bad place, ouch. You either will just give up and eat because you don't have the desperation for the spiritual backup you need or, if you do get through it, you'll just regain the weight and be right back in the same spot. There's nothing wrong with wanting to drop a few pounds. And if you actually Not Eat and pray instead, you will lose weight. I lost a total of 50 pounds over 13 months and kept 30 pounds off permanently.

So what I'm trying to say is if you do this you will lose weight and look better, but that should be an awesome added bonus and not your goal. I had tried and failed many many times to lose weight and keep it off. But when I stopped eating and started crying out for real help, the weight just came off without any real effort focused on it. And stayed off.

EAT YOUR VEGETABLES!

If you want to keep weight off, or look healthier, or feel better physically in your joints or whatever else ails you, then there is something I can tell you here, from the Bible, that works like magic. There is only one catch: it may be harder than Not Eating at all.

You may have heard about or even tried this thing called the Daniel plan or the Daniel fast, or the Daniel whatever. It's almost a little cottage industry now. But you don't need to go subscribe to the Columbia House eight track Daniel plan monthly installments of stuff coming to the house to help. Basically it's just a way of eating that can improve your health. Problem is, there's two different diet descriptions in the book of Daniel.

One is where Daniel is mourning and for three weeks he doesn't eat any meat or rich food, or drink wine, or use any smell-good stuff. And the second description of a way of eating is at the beginning of the book. When Daniel and his buds are chosen to begin a three-year period of studying to serve in the king's palace, they are to be put on the Kings diet of delicacies and wine. But Daniel opts out of this eating arrangement, and his group eats only vegetables and drinks only water.

After ten days, they look better and healthier than the other students who are the King's diet. So they were allowed to eat that way throughout their training. Their training was for three years.

So that's only vegetables and water for 3 years, people. At the end of that time they were ten times more capable than the others. They looked better. They had more wisdom. And they had an unusual aptitude for understanding.

Because of this ultimate grooviness they were promoted to the top right away. So if you want earned success in your field, If you want to be trim and fit, if you want to be wise and smart, then once you are finished with this Not Eating to free your captives, you can try eating like Daniel. Vegetables and water. Only. He did it for three years. When he started, he was one of the captives. At the end, he was a close adviser to the king.

We did this all vegetable diet once too, for 21 days. It takes planning and preparation like you would not believe. If you're Not Eating, all you have to do is Not Eat. But if you're eating only vegetables, I mean only vegetables, and it's 1 PM like on that one day I walked into a 7-Eleven hungry and realized, there is nothing in this entire store that I can eat. I am surrounded by food and I cannot eat any of it. So you have to plan ahead. Also, to eat only vegetables, you have to drop your culturally ingrained ideas of what is breakfast food. You're just going to eat vegetables at every meal, and breakfast is really just the first meal of the day, so get over it.

Potato chips are not vegetables. Don't be a tool.

Find and buy some vegetables you can just eat raw, like little bags of baby carrots. If you go out to a restaurant, just get a salad with vinegar dressing and no added sugar. Figure it out. If you want to lose weight, keep off the weight, be smarter, look younger, and get promoted faster, this is a way to do it. You can work out the details as you go along.

That right there is your whole diet plan. Do it as long as you can and as often. It will also change the way you eat for the times you're not actually on the diet. I'm not claiming I'm the World's Cleanest Eater, but my regular way of eating is so much healthier than before. Shoot I almost took my shirt off the last time I went running on the beach. I said almost. Don't be scared. You can try this diet After you try Not Eating. Because, remember, you are going to Not Eat for something way more important than weight loss.

WHAT'S YOUR PROBLEM?!

You haven't really heard the real good news yet. Which is how this is going to help YOU. So far it seems like it's just about Not doing something. Something that's critical to life itself. How to Not Eat sounds very Old Testament-like, doesn't it?

But really this book, this idea, this thing that you are going to try, finally, is about what YOU are going to get. Why would you Not Eat? What in the world are you trying to do by Not Eating?

The Bible, Old and New Testament, is the best place to go for an amazing collection of stories about Not Eating and praying and the miracles that follow. Success stories. Pretty much every story of a person or people responding to a problem by Not Eating and asking for Divine Intervention ends up with the Divine Intervention. The problem is zapped and goes away (with a little work from you of course), time after time.

Why are you considering Not Eating? There could be countless reasons why you might just be desperate enough to try it. Let's look at some of the big reasons and maybe look at some of the examples of people who have Not Eaten when faced with those kinds of big problems.

Maybe their victories are about to become yours.

WAMMO!

Maybe you've got so many things going wrong, so many enemies - physical or spiritual - chasing you, that you think its the End. Literally. Somebody's going to die. Or everything's going to blow up. Or both. That was me. I was going to die. And everyone around me was in serious danger.

Then I read the Book of Esther.

I first learned about fasting from the book of Esther, you may recall, in the Old Testament. I had never even heard of it. The book of Esther that is. But it seemed to come at me from every direction until finally I would just try it. What I did not tell you earlier about the king saving Esther and her people was their enemy got impaled on a pole that he had meant for her peoples harm. And then the Jews were given authority to go chop off the heads of all people who meant them harm. It's a real action-thriller of a book, right there in the Bible.

Just as a reminder, Esther did not fast alone. She enlisted help from her friends and family. She got them to fast with her. If the trouble is deep enough, you may have to do this too. Esther volunteered to Not Eat and then got the others to Not Eat with her, and they were saved. They were all going to be executed and instead they got positions of power. They got to kill their enemies. And they all lived happily ever after. They chopped off some heads, took no plunder, and then had a huge feast. Like Jewish Pirates. Boss Jewish Pirates.

In this first example of fasting from the Bible, they were not trying to be free from one thing, rather their entire lives were at stake. The situation looked hopeless. They had no power. The decisions had all been made. All they could do was Not Eat and go to their king. To literally save them.

And, as we will see over and over and over again, it worked. This worked in my life as you know now. I was a dang mess. And now I'm just a little messy. Again, I didn't have some great faith when I started. I really didn't have much of a choice. For some reason, I could not turn around without getting some story or book or word or person telling me about fasting fasting fasting until I thought I'm either crazy or I'm going to do it. I really didn't have any choice: if you're getting squished down by the thumb of the Almighty, you don't really have a choice. So I did like the book said, and I got a similar outcome as in the book. It was like God himself looked down and listened to the groans of a doomed man and then reached in and opened up the doors of my death cell and set me free.

Literally.

So if you have problems that look like they are never going to get better, they can actually get better. If you gather your people like Esther did - and like i did - and Not Eat together. Maybe God will save you like He saved the Jews. And the Basses.

WAIT THERE'S MORE!

Esther and Mordecai did one more thing you'll be super excited about. Because of how awesome it all turned out in their favor, they set aside regular times of Not Eating to be followed in the future, just like they had regular times of celebration. See, aren't you super excited? That's right: they decided if they were going to have set times for good times, they should also plan out dates when they just would Not Eat.

A time to cheer and a time to lament. So maybe you should think about investing yourself in a little denial now and then, even if life is just going along normally. The Book of Ecclesiastes says that's a good thing. So did Esther and Mordecai, two Not Eating Ninjas from The Scrolls.

I do it. Sometimes it's just until dinner. Sometimes it's a whole day. It's way harder to Not Eat when things are going pretty good. But I'm always glad afterward. You are never going to finish a fast and say Wow that was a mistake.

Repeat: You are never going to regret Not Eating. Once you are done, you will be so glad you did it. So don't quit before your time is up. Endings are better than beginnings. It says that in Ecclesiastes too. You may want to mark the days on a calendar, or you may want to just do it every so often - whatever works for you. This is not a collection of rules; it is a guide to your better life.

RIPPED UP LIKE A DUECE!

Maybe life, without warning, has just knocked you the heck out. You're just walking along, singing a song, and then ka-bloooey! The Big One hits. Your arm falls off, or you get the cancer, or you're in a big wreck, or your kid gets kicked out of school, or you - fill in the dang blank from your own dang life. Whatever it is, you were groovy one second, and then the next second you were definitely not groovy.

This kind of thing happened to a guy named Saul in the Book of Acts in the New Testament of the Bible. Saul had a powerful job and tons of influence. He wasn't the coolest of dudes, mind you, but he thought he was kicking bass and taking names. He and his buds were cruising down the road, looking for some Jesus-followers to whack, and then out of nowhere Saul got struck by lightning - is what it looked like - and he heard a voice from the sky. When his friends tried to help him up, they discovered he been knocked completely sightless, blinded by the Light.

So you know what Saul did? He did Not Eat for three days, that's what he did. After that, some guy came over and prayed for him. And Saul's sight was restored. He got baptized, started going by the name

Paul, and immediately changed the direction of his life. He had been a chief persecutor of believers in the new faith, but he became the most influential follower of Jesus who ever lived. He ended up writing a good portion of what is now the New Testament.

So not only was his sight restored but he was transformed from a mean little hater to man whose true descriptions of love are so powerful that they're used in the majority of weddings today, 2000 years later, on the other side of the world.

Love is patient, love is kind. It does not envy, it does not boast, it is not proud. It does not dishonor others, it is not self-seeking, it is not easily angered, it keeps no record of wrongs. Love does not delight in evil but rejoices with the truth. It always protects, always trusts, always hopes, always perseveres.

Love never fails.

That is what you call an underdog story and everybody loves an underdog. Blind Saul became St. Paul.

So if you just got smacked down, and you want to be the underdog who pulls off the miracle comeback, start your journey by Stopping Eating.

SMH!

Maybe you have an affliction that just won't go away, even though you have prayed and prayed and called on prayer circles and prayer warriors and had hands laid on and... and and Nothing happens. It just keeps plaguing you. Maybe even gets worse. Maybe you go to church and tithe and rescue kittens and the whole mess, but you never get the cure.

This kind can only come out by prayer and fasting.

There was a boy in Jesus's day who was plagued his whole life by violent fits. The boy's father brought him to Jesus's disciples, who had been healing people. But they couldn't heal the boy. Then Jesus showed up, and the boy's father told Him what had happened. Jesus looked at his peeps and said: how long am I going to have to put up with you generation of bozos?

Then Jesus straight up healed the boy in the middle of one of his fits, and everyone was amazed. Of course. Later his disciples asked Jesus why He could do what they could not do. "This kind can only come out by prayer and fasting." Was what He said.

This I know from experience: some problems – call them personal demons if you want – can plague you your whole life and never get better no matter what you try. If you believe in Jesus you may have tried a couple of things over and over and over with no success: calling on the name of Jesus in prayer and reading his word. If those things haven't worked, you may have to Not Eat to be free.

There's been problems I could not shake no matter how much I prayed or read the Bible. But then I fasted and they disappeared. Some never to return. Some creeped back a little and I had to fast again. But either way, they went away. They came out by prayer and fasting. Before they had just sat there and uncle festered.

If you'd rather live with your problems than live a little while without food, then just go on set this book down and walk away. But you can also try just not putting food in your food hole to see if the problem comes out. I say go for it. You got nothing to lose but a pound or two. But you just might get a freedom you had long ago given up on getting.

One thing to note here is that Jesus did not go fast and then come back to heal the boy. He must have already been fasted up. Remember Esther and Mordecai setting aside regular times for Not Eating? If you do that, which it appears that Jesus did, you'll be ready for problems ahead of time that can only be dealt with by prayer and fasting. You'll be all fasted up, like Jesus was.

Just know that Not Eating worked for Jesus and the boy with fits. And it worked for me, Greg Bass, so it can work for anybody.

Is there something in your life that just will not get better no matter how much you pray or read the bible? Do you really want to get better? Then put down your fork and pick up the Book and see what happens.

KNOCK IT OFF!

Maybe, just maybe, you have been doing some bad stuff. It might not be as bad as other people's bad stuff, but you know it ain't right. And it says in the Book that if you do stuff that's kinda bad and you know it's kinda bad and you do it anyway, you may be worse off than somebody who does something way More Badder but doesn't know it's bad. Maybe you didn't even realize how wrong it was but now you do. There's many ways to soft shoe this discussion about how you may have been walking a rocky road to trouble town. I did a whole heck of a lot of that kind of nonsense myself. So I know all about it. It's not too late for you to get to your happy place. Here's why:

The story of Jonah is pretty awesome. It's actually an entire book in the Bible. A four chapter, two page book. A two page book used to seem like a ridiculous concept before the Internet. But now I'm thinking: Do I really have 10 minutes to read a book?

So you know the story of Jonah right? God told Jonah to go to the city of Ninevah and tell them that He was ticked off at them for their violence and evil ways. But Jonah got on a ship going the opposite direction. Now you shouldn't say no way jose to the Creator of the Universe.

God sent a big storm and the sailors found out why and threw that Jonah into the cold cold sea. Where he got swallowed up by a big fish. Jonah lived in the belly of that whale or whatever it was for three days. While he was in there, Jonah sincerely said sorry to the Lord and then got spit out on shore. There's something about getting thrown overboard and swallowed by a creature of the deep that will tend to turn your mind to the Lord, let me tell you.

I used to not believe the Bible, in part because of how certain people told me I had to believe stories like Jonah were basically a historical reporting of facts. So now I just read it for myself. Turns out, for whatever else it is that I don't want to debate here, the Bible is also most definitely an awesome book about what goes on in your mind, man. The Bible is not just some history book about Jonah, the unluckiest of the Hebrews. It is about your heart. It is about how you think. Today. If Jesus is the Word then this word is about what's happening in your temple right now.

The book of Jonah is also about these people who lived in this city called Nineveh. And they were not living right. God sent Jonah to warn them. Jonah ran the other way. The fish swallowed him up and spit him out. And only then did Jonah go to Ninevah to warn them that God was ticked off.

And here's the cool thing: here's what this violent, evil people of Ninevah did: the King proclaimed a fast for everyone in the city, from highest to lowest. Even including the animals. Even the puppies. They repented in their hearts but also in their actions. I mean, that is really putting on the brakes hard when a whole city stops eating to pray.

And God saw them. And they were saved. All of them. Doom turned to Joy.

Maybe you need to stop eating and call on God because you've been doing wrong. You've heard that bad things can happen to good people? Well bad things can happen to bad people, too, and way more often. And way worse. Maybe you're not bad people, but you just got off track somehow and now you're way down the wrong road.

Stop Eating. Pray.

Who knows? Maybe God will display His awesome mercy one more time. Maybe this time, just for you.

The other part of this story is Jonah not doing what he knew for a fact that the Lord wanted him to do. Every time I put off writing this book, I saw Jonah. So that is why I am passing on this message. I know I'm supposed to. I can only hope and pray that y'all or all y'all or some of y'all take it heart and start Not Eating and see if the Lord Himself puts your life on the good foot.

WHAT THE?

There's going to be times in your life when you get bad news. And sometimes the news is going to be really bad. What are you going to do? How will you respond when you find out? If you're a smoker, maybe you will smoke it up. If you're a drinker, maybe you will drink it down. If you're a hot head, maybe you'll Break out in fisticuffs. If you're depressed, maybe you will just lay down.

You also might be living in the fallout of someone else's sins. Maybe one of your parents or grandparents did something stupid and you have to clean up the mess. Or maybe they passed down their mess to you and now you are doing the same dang dumb stuff they did. Well you are in luck. Read on.

There was a guy named Nehemiah in the book of Nehemiah - go figure - who got some really bad news. His people back in Jerusalem had been trampled by invaders. The walls around the city were in rubble, and the gates were burned, and the people were living unprotected in squalor, open to more attacks, but with nothing left to lose. It was, as they say, a bad deal. But the story behind the story is that the previous generations who had lived in Jerusalem had decided to let it all hang out. They abandoned the good path and started partying hard. And guess what? Stuff happened. Eventually they got handed over to their enemies and the walls came down.

Here's what Nehemiah did: he Stopped Eating and prayed to God for days when he heard. So he got really bad news, and his response was to Stop Eating and start praying. Then he made a plan to deal with the problem, while he was still Not Eating, and prayed this plan would be successful. Then, and only then, did Nehemiah take action.

It's important to see the way he prayed I think. Not so you can use it as a magic formulary to get what you want from God (Who is not, you might be surprised to find out, the Magic Santy Clause in the sky). Either God is made up or God is real. And if God is real, He will not be manipulated by me or you or any other puny little human.

But if God is real, you better approach Him with a humble heart. Nehemiah prayed this way: Great and awesome God, please hear my prayers to you night and day, confessing the sins of my people, including me and my ancestors. We've treated you like dirt. I'm turning to you and asking you to redeem us.

Try modeling that prayer, from your heart, and see what happens. Notice that Nehemiah also prayed for forgiveness of the sins of his ancestors, even though he was going to have to clean up their mess.

If you want God to be with you as you tackle a huge problem, you can Stop Eating before you make your request. God seems to honor that again and again and those old books and scrolls. And God will honor it In your current life too. I'm not going to lay out all my personal problems here that God graciously handled for me. This book is about how you - YOU - can get God to handle your problems by you Not Eating.

Nehemiah didn't just Not Eat and pray and then everything got immediately better. That's just what he did in the first page or two of the book. There's a whole story that follows of all the Work that went into the rebuilding. He had challenges while fixing the problem. Rebuilding the walls and gates was a huge job, and their enemies were many. He asked God to help during those challenges, and so he overcame them. The wall around Jerusalem was rebuilt and all the gates restored. But there were still battles.

Sometimes your problems might just go poof and disappear, but way more times you are going to have get up, get busy, and do the work. Only then, as you work, you might have the Lord's blessing. And that is all you will need.

So don't be discouraged if you Don't Eat and pray instead, and your problem is still there. Keep trying. Keep working. Why do you think we fasted for 100 days in a year? Because life was all good at the Bass House? Heck no. Do you think I'm nuts? Oh yeah, I just love Not Eating for weeks on end, over and over.

No, I kept Not Eating because I still had many challenges. I saw just enough miracles to keep doing it. Nehemiah and his rebuild crew came under attack after attack. Even after Not Eating and getting the King's blessing and help. They slept in their clothes to be on guard. They kept one hand on their swords at all time. The other on a hammer. But they didn't quit.

So don't expect Easy Street just because you Don't Eat. But Do expect victory. Eventual victory.

And check this out. After Jerusalem was rebuilt they had a big feast and read God's word and had a huge celebration. And guess what they did? The people all got together and... They fasted! That's right. They Stopped Eating and repented of all their previous bologna together. They committed to changing their ways.

So when you Not Eat and God sweeps your problems away, you may want to respond by Not Eating again, so you don't go back to whatever was causing the problems the first time. This all may sound kind of sucky, because it is kind of sucky. But remember, the story started with the whole people being run over and run down and hopeless. And then one person fasted for them. And the story ends with rebuilt lives in a rebuilt town and great celebrations.

If you are trying to rebuild your walls after a big mess of your own creation, you might take the time to see if you are just recreating some bad behaviors passed down to you from one of your ancestors. Maybe you lie to your woman because your dad ran out on your mom. Or maybe you can't commit to a relationship because your mom was a floozy. Or maybe you smoke crack because your granny was a crackhead. It's a big world, who knows? But in any case maybe you should try praying for the forgiveness of your ancestors when you are Not Eating. It might set you free from some rusty old chains. We did it. It went a long way to stop us from walking down those old roads.

So if that's what you want, maybe you need to do the Nehemiah for your people. Maybe you need to Not Eat. If you've come under some attack and your walls are down and your people have lost hope, now at least you know what to do first.

GOING TO CALIFORNIA

Maybe you are going out on a journey, or starting a new chapter in your life, or taking some risk that's necessary to get where you're going. Maybe you are getting married. Or going back to school. Or taking a new job. Or moving across the country. Or starting a business. Maybe you've got to go home and you're afraid there's going to be trouble. Homecomings often are fraught with danger. You can stop eating and petition God to help you.

That's what happened in the book of Ezra. Ezra was heading back to Jerusalem and the trip was fraught with peril. He was leading his people, and they were carrying valuables right through enemy territory. (Your enemies might not be the kind hiding in the hills with masks but they can still be just as real, even if they're hiding in your heart.) Ezra did not want to ask the king for help and protection on this journey, because he had already told the king that the gracious hand of God would protect them. God will take care of us, is what he had already said. But instead of just being an old windbag going on about the Lord, as some people do, Ezra actually did something.

Talk is cheap. Talk about God is even cheaper. Ezra put his money where his mouth was by not putting food where his mouth was. He proclaimed a fast among the traveling group before they headed out. As a group, they did Not Eat. They asked God to help them. And God answered their prayers.

Their trip was safe and successful through the badlands, even though they were loaded down with gold and polished bronze. God honored their Not Eating. If you have a dangerous or risky or uncertain journey ahead, Don't Eat before hand and pray for safety instead. Especially if you've been bragging about trusting God, you better trust God when the time comes.

Don't be a windbag, set down the feedbag.

Like Ezra, you might need to Not Eat because you're going on a journey, be it physical or metaphorical. If you Stop Eating, you set yourself up to receive some supernatural help from a source who's help really means something. Google maps can give you directions, but the God of heaven can offer you his protection. Jesus is way more powerful than Pedro.

It might seem crazy that I'm offering all these claims about good things happening in such a wide variety of situations all By Just Not Eating. But remember these two things: each of these examples is from the Bible, not me. And my wife and I have tried all of these ourselves, and it's changed our lives. For the better - the way better.

BIG BAD WOLF

I'm almost afraid to relay this next story about Not Eating because it either might seem too hard to comprehend or too unbelievable to think it's anything more than a metaphor. But the story behind the story is more important than the number in the story. Please keep reading.

One of the most amazing things that can happen to you if you Don't Eat is it can give you the ability to withstand temptations. Even and especially temptations that have ruined you in the past. Your specific temptations. Can become powerless over you.

You might be tempted by sex. Or drugs. Or rock and roll. But temptations are just as often on the inside, your inside. You might be tempted to run and hide. You might be tempted to lie. You might be to feel jealous. You might be tempted to lash out or lie down and quit. You might be tempted to hold on to wrongs. The list goes on.

If you have some knowledge of the Bible, you might have heard about Jesus's forty day fast in the wilderness. That may be the only fast you know of. It might even seem metaphorical. But it definitely might have kept you from thinking fasting is something for you. Let's check it out.

Jesus, like you, was tempted. All that Jesus did in the Bible, all his public works that were recorded and then changed every thing that followed, began as soon as he was baptized. Jesus comes out of the water, baptized, and the very next thing recorded is Jesus being led by the spirit to be tempted. And he doesn't eat. For forty days. And for forty nights. And it says he was hungry. Duh.

And guess what? At the end of the forty days, the very first temptation was to turns some stones into bread and eat them. Mmmm bread. Because if Jesus was really the son of God, then He could do that. He could turn stones into bread and eat them. And no matter who he was, bread after 40 days would be delicious.

Except Jesus had a word for the tempter instead. Man doesn't live by bread alone, but by every word that comes from the mouth of God. (That's in the Old Scrolls) So He didn't fall to the temptation. He countered with The Word.

First of all don't be freaked out by the forty day thing. Jesus was about to be tempted to rule the world rather than save it. The stakes were pretty high, you could say. You probably don't have to quit eating for forty days. Probably.

Each time Jesus was tempted in that story, he had the exact right word from The Word as an answer to the temptation. My temptations aren't the same as Jesus' temptations. Neither are yours. That's why it's important to spend your extra time while you're Not Eating reading from the Bible, and then to continue doing that as you begin eating again.

Praying is good, but it's mostly you talking. You want God to talk to you, to give you the words you will need. Let Him write His words on your heart, so you will have them when you are face-to-face with your tempter.

Jesus resisted his temptations with the word of God three times. Then the tempter went away and left him alone. Then angels came down and attended to Him. This is great news. You don't have to resist forever. Don't Eat, pray, read the word, use it to resist your temptations, and your temptations will leave you alone. Finally. You won't have to fight and struggle over and over, forever and ever, amen. You can get free. Angels will take care of you, somehow. Don't ask me. And you'll be able to eat again, but with a peace and freedom you couldn't ever imagine before.

Stop worrying about how long you are not going to eat. Start believing you can finally resist the devil and he will flee. Get Behind Me Satan is not just an awesome album by The White Stripes, FYI.

Since you cannot be tempted to turn stones into bread, because you're not God, then you can't use the words Jesus used in order to resist your temptations. You have to get a clue what your real temptations are first. This will happen while you're fasting. Then you have to get words from the Word of God that you can use to rebuke your temptations. The miracle is you can get words from the Bible specifically to repel your temptations. And these words will have real power because they are not just words.

But not if you just sit there with the book closed.

TAKE THIS JOB AND SHOVE IT!

Maybe you're just ready to give up. Maybe you've been living right, trying to do the right thing, living a life of integrity, and yet you keep coming under attack. You hit opposition at every turn. You may even have enemies trying to track you down when all you've done is what God wanted you to do.

Maybe you are saying to God I've had enough! I can't take it anymore! I just got to lay down and quit.

That's what happened to Elijah, one of the great prophets and heroes of the Old Testament. Elijah had become afraid and discouraged because the king's people were out to kill him once again. Elijah felt like he was the only one left fighting the good fight, and now the bad guys in power were coming for him too. And like no matter what he did, people didn't listen, didn't change. So he might as well bounce.

That's usually what happened with the prophets: people tried to kill them. If you read those old scrolls, you'll find the words most often heard from God are: Don't be afraid. Don't be discouraged. Yet here was this great hero of the Israelites, afraid and discouraged.

"Take my life!" He called out to the Lord. Maybe that's you. If so, do what Elijah did. He Stopped Eating – Surprise – and went to an isolated place to listen carefully for direction from God. While he was there in the cave, waiting on God, a heavy wind ripped through, shattering rocks. But God wasn't in the wind. And then an earthquake shook the ground. But God wasn't in the earthquake. And then a wildfire tore up the land. But God wasn't in the fire. But after the fire there was a quiet whisper. God was whispering to Elijah. And God comforted him and gave him new direction and strength. So Elijah went back out into the world to complete his mission.

Remember, that Bible is not just a life and times history of Elijah, it is The Creator speaking to you, if you will listen, about your life. Now. If it was only a Hebrew history text then big whoop. The world is full of history books. And I love history, but still. And it's not just a metaphor. There is something real for you today.

Sometimes you can get all caught up in the noise from the world and your own thoughts, so much that you can't hear the encouraging whisper from the Lord. If you're serious about wanting to hear what God says, you might have to put in some effort. You might have to Not Eat first. And if you then get a whisper from the creator of the universe, you're getting something good.

And if you are ready to just pack it in, remember what God says most: Don't be afraid. Don't be discouraged.

So don't give up. Just give up food. Not Eat and pray. Then listen quietly. Maybe, just maybe, God will whisper to you. Don't be afraid. Don't be discouraged. And for a while, Don't be Eating.

SIRI, TAKE ME TO THE PROMISED LAND

Maybe you feel like you been wandering around, lost in the desert in your life. You just can't get anywhere. You feel like you're going in circles. Tired and worn out, and you'd like nothing better than to rest at the feet of a loving father who would love you and protect you and help you get where you are going.

Moses did that. In the book of Exodus, Moses was leading the Jews through the desert in their long trip from slavery to the promised land. What should have been a short trip was taking a lifetime. Literally. Everyone was fed up and they started doing their own thing and even wishing they could go back to their old lives of slavery.

They were lost, physically, geographically, and spiritually. But Moses got to go be in the presence of God. And while he was in the presence of the Lord, Moses fasted for 40 days. Like there was God, and there was Moses. I could almost understand the Not Eating for 40 days thing, probably, if I could get the smallest glimpse of what it's like to be in the presence of God. But I can't. Not yet.

But here is what I do know: if you want to be closer to God, in real terms – I mean really feel close to the creator of the heavens and earth – you can try Not Eating. Just don't try it for too long or you'll actually be meeting Him face-to-face. Ha ha that is a lame fasting joke. The kind you'll hear from people all the time if you tell them you're fasting. Which you should not do. But it's okay for me because I'm writing the dang book urging you to do it.

During Moses's Not Eating time, God carved the 10 Commandments on two stone tablets. You may have heard of them. They're kind of a big deal. If you Stop Eating and try to sit at the feet of the Lord, he may give you some pretty good insight too.

The very first commandment, by the Way, is to have no other gods before me, says God. You may think that's pretty easy right? Just avoid being a Hindu or worshiping a Redwood or something. But what if it means don't make anything more important than God in you heart? Like food. Or Sunday football.

What if you can make food into a god? Thinking about it all the time, getting your comfort from it, looking to it to give your life meaning? Kind of sounds like a god doesn't it? I don't mean just enjoying eating, because that can be a real blessing. God says it's a good thing in Ecclesiastes to enjoy a good meal. But, on the other hand, how many rooms in your house are dedicated full-time or half-time to food? How many to God? Me too. I'm only asking okay?

So what if by Not Eating for a while you can ensure that you don't make eating first in your life? What if by Not Eating you are making space for God to come in and give you a real sense of peace? I looked for peace in the bottom of every carton of ice cream many times, friends. Didn't find it. Desert and dessert are only one letter off.

But what if you just want to get out of the dang desert? You can still have your mac & cheese later. But nothing beats knowing that God is with you. And you might need to be like Moses and Not Eat for a while to find this out for yourself.

If you can't where you want to go in your life, if you're running in circles, maybe you just need to stop trying so hard to get there and start trying to get a little bit more in the presence of God. Maybe the best way to do that Stop Eating and seek Him out during that time. Worked out for Moses and his peeps. Might work out for you, too.

NOTHING TO SEE HERE

Maybe you have kids who've lived their whole lives with you and and are now about to leave home to go to college or wherever. Or maybe you are about to leave your current life yourself and embark on something new, and you are not sure which direction to take. Or maybe you are going to help choose a new church leader, or sales manager or shift leader and you want to make the right choice, but you're not sure how. Or maybe there's a change coming up in your family or friends that's going to be hard to handle.

In the Book of Acts, Paul and Barnabas are shown to be Not Eating and praying a couple of times. One time was with a group of church leaders and the holy spirit showed up and told the group that Paul and Barnabas were to go on a special mission. This is when they first went out into the world to talk about Jesus.

So during a fast, the Holy Spirit gave them the big mission for the rest of their lives. And told them about it. When they started the fast, they were just a couple of dudes. When they ended the fast, they were heading out to become the most important missionaries of all time.

During another fast later, they were appointing elders to a church before moving on to another city. Before they did this, they prayed and fasted, asking the Lord to guide the people they were leaving behind. They were no longer going to be with these people so they left them with the best thing they had: blessings from God. Before they split, they spent time Not Eating and praying because, after that, they would not be there to give the newly appointed elders advice or correction or encouragement face-to-face.

In fact, before they picked the new leaders they were going to leave in charge, they fasted so they would make the right choice. Can you imagine how many better leaders we would have, how many fewer creeps, if those in charge would Not Eat and pray instead before they made the choice?

During our time of Not Eating, our sons were graduating high school and leaving home to go to college. They had lived with us their whole life, and now they were going to be living someplace else. So before they left home we Stopped Eating. And prayed. And committed them to the Lord. My wife sent our sons out in the world by handing them over to the Lord in prayer.

And the Lord has been with our sons. And also with my wife. Not eating lessened the power of the emotions that would come during that time. Because there is power in committing a person the Lord when they're embarking on a big adventure, or starting a position of leadership, or going to college. And that power is intensified by Not Eating first. God takes note.

But there's also freedom for those doing the committing, if they will fast before they pray. It's not always just impending doom or lingering pressure that can be relieved by Not Eating. Sometimes even if the change is good and right, it is good to be preceded by Not Eating. Not Eating food isn't just some horrible time of self-denial, it's opening your life up to a power greater than what's under your control. Immensely greater. And awesomeness may follow.

Maybe the Lord has great plans for you that He will make clear if you will take some time to Not Eat and seek direction.

Your uneasiness about a change coming is because you don't know the future. And you can't control it either. But you want it to go good and right. Well this whole Not Eating adventure is based on the idea that you might just get help from a God who does know the future and can control it. A little faith won't hurt you. It may just save you.

THIS WILL ONLY HURT A LITTLE

Do you want to make sure you are doing this right? I mean you don't want to Not Eat and have it be for nothing. Do you want to finally be free because God Himself will come to save you? Then check this out.

The last fast. And a warning from God. Yes. To me and possibly to you. And a promise too. There's a book called Isaiah in the Old Testament, the ancient scrolls. I suggest you read it. It's important to note that Paul wrote in the Bible that the old scrolls are not what God says about other people but instead what God says to us - that's me and you. Not those other people. So if you read this book of Isaiah you should probably be asking: what does this say about me? Then things will get really interesting.

In chapter 58, God is using the prophet Isaiah to speak out to these rebellious Jews (they were so, so bad – like an entire race of teenagers).

The Jews are like, Hey padre we are fasting her people, we are humbling ourselves and seeking you out, and you're not doing anything for us. What the heck? God himself says this: you think fasting is about coming before me and being all sorry and full of regret, then going and doing the same thing over and over? It ain't. You're still fighting with each other, and taking advantage of each other, and punching and hollering, and you want me to come help you just because you're Not Eating?

So we're starting to see a glimpse here that an absence of food in your face doesn't equal God in your heart. It's not a magic trick you control.

God tells them what to do when they fast: Free the Captives. Loose the chains of injustice. Break every chain. Feed the hungry. Shelter the poor. Clothe the naked. Don't turn away from your own flesh and blood. Do these things, and I will come running to your rescue when you call. Don't just stop eating, he says. Stop pointing fingers of blame at each other. Stop talking maliciously about one another. Do away with your yolks of oppression.

Then your light will break free like the dawn and your healing will quickly appear.

Make your fast about changing you and your light will rise in the darkness, your midnight will shine like the noonday sun.

The Lord will be there to guide you and He'll satisfy your needs in the sun-scorched land. You will be like a well watered garden, like a spring whose waters never fail.

Your people will rebuild the ancient ruins. You will be called the repairer of broken walls. The restorer of streets and homes.

Then when you call, the Lord will answer.

'Yes, I am here,' he will quickly reply.

For the mouth of the Lord has spoken.

Amen.

Not Eating stories mentioned in this book:

Esther 4-5

Esther 9

Jonah 3

Matthew 4

Matthew 6

Ezra 8

Nehemiah 1

1 Kings 19

Exodus 34

Acts 9

Acts 13

Acts 14

Isaiah 58

Mark 9

Daniel 1